Living with Progressive Supranuclear Palsy: A Guide to Symptom Management

Laura Louizos

Table of Contents

Chapter 5: Cognitive and Behavioral Changes

- Identifying Cognitive Symptoms
- Strategies for Managing Behavioral Changes
- Cognitive Stimulation Activities
- Support for Emotional Well-being

Chapter 6: Managing Pain and Discomfort

- Understanding Sources of Pain in PSP
- Pain Relief Strategies
- Complementary Therapies
- Medications for Pain Management

Chapter 7: Daily Living and Practical Tips

- Adapting the Home Environment
- Establishing Routines and Schedules
- Tips for Personal Care and Hygiene
- Assistive Devices and Technology

Chapter 8: Nutrition and Diet

- Importance of Nutrition in PSP
- Dietary Recommendations
- Managing Weight and Nutritional Intake
- Meal Planning and Preparation Tips

Chapter 9: Emotional and Psychological Support

- Coping with the Diagnosis
- Managing Stress and Anxiety
- Support for Caregivers
- Counseling and Support Groups

Introduction

Understanding Progressive Supranuclear Palsy (PSP)

Progressive Supranuclear Palsy (PSP) is a rare, degenerative neurological disorder that affects movement, balance, vision, speech, and swallowing. PSP is often misdiagnosed due to its similarities with other neurodegenerative diseases like Parkinson's disease and Alzheimer's disease. Understanding PSP can be challenging for both individuals diagnosed with the condition and their caregivers due to its complex and varied symptoms.

PSP typically manifests in mid to late adulthood, and while the exact cause is unknown, it is believed to be related to the accumulation of a protein called tau in the brain. This accumulation leads to the gradual deterioration of brain cells in areas that control movement and other vital functions. The progression of PSP varies from person to person, making it essential to have a comprehensive understanding of the condition and its management.

Purpose of the Book

"Living with Progressive Supranuclear Palsy: A Guide to Symptom Management" aims to provide a thorough, practical, and compassionate resource for individuals diagnosed with PSP and their caregivers. This book is designed to:

- Offer clear, accessible information about PSP, its symptoms, and progression.
- Present effective strategies for managing the wide range of symptoms associated with PSP.
- Provide practical tips and tools for daily living to improve the quality of life for those affected by PSP.
- Address the emotional and psychological challenges that come with a PSP diagnosis, offering support and coping strategies.

- Share personal stories and experiences from individuals living with PSP and their caregivers to foster a sense of community and shared understanding.
- Highlight resources, support networks, and further reading to empower individuals and caregivers with the knowledge they need to navigate this journey.

How to Use This Guide

This book is organized into chapters, each focusing on a specific aspect of PSP and its management. Whether you are newly diagnosed, a long-term caregiver, or a healthcare professional seeking more information, you can use this guide in several ways:

- **Read from Start to Finish:** For a comprehensive understanding of PSP and its management, read the book sequentially.
- **Focus on Specific Chapters:** If you are looking for information on a particular symptom or area of concern, refer to the relevant chapter directly.
- **Use as a Reference:** Keep this book on hand as a reference guide to revisit as new symptoms or challenges arise.
- **Share with Others:** This guide can be shared with family members, friends, and healthcare providers to help them understand PSP and provide better support.

Living with PSP is undoubtedly challenging, but with the right information, support, and resources, it is possible to manage symptoms effectively and maintain a good quality of life. This book aims to be a trusted companion on this journey, offering hope, practical advice, and a sense of community to everyone affected by PSP.

Chapter 1: Overview of PSP

What is Progressive Supranuclear Palsy (PSP)?

Progressive Supranuclear Palsy (PSP) is a rare, degenerative brain disorder that impairs movement, balance, speech, vision, and thinking. Named for its hallmark characteristic of supranuclear gaze palsy—difficulty moving the eyes up and down—PSP is often mistaken for other neurodegenerative conditions like Parkinson's disease, leading to challenges in early and accurate diagnosis.

PSP falls under the category of tauopathies, which are conditions associated with the abnormal accumulation of the tau protein in the brain. This build-up leads to the deterioration of cells in areas crucial for controlling movement and cognitive functions.

Causes and Risk Factors

The exact cause of PSP is not yet known. However, researchers believe that a combination of genetic, environmental, and possibly lifestyle factors contribute to its development. Unlike some neurodegenerative diseases, PSP does not appear to have a strong hereditary component, though certain genetic variations may increase susceptibility.

Factors believed to influence PSP include:

- **Age:** Most commonly, PSP affects individuals in their 60s and 70s.
- **Gender:** Men are slightly more likely to develop PSP than women.
- **Genetics:** While rare, some genetic mutations have been linked to PSP.

- **Environmental Factors:** Exposure to certain toxins or chemicals may increase risk, though more research is needed in this area.

Symptoms and Progression

PSP symptoms can vary widely among individuals but generally include the following:

1. **Motor Symptoms:**
   - **Postural Instability and Falls:** Difficulty maintaining balance, often resulting in unexplained falls.
   - **Bradykinesia:** Slowness of movement.
   - **Rigidity:** Muscle stiffness, particularly in the neck and upper body.
   - **Dystonia:** Abnormal muscle contractions leading to twisted postures.
2. **Eye Movement Abnormalities:**
   - **Supranuclear Gaze Palsy:** Difficulty moving the eyes up and down.
   - **Blurred or Double Vision:** Due to impaired coordination of eye movements.
3. **Speech and Swallowing Difficulties:**
   - **Dysarthria:** Slurred or slow speech.
   - **Dysphagia:** Difficulty swallowing, leading to choking or aspiration.
4. **Cognitive and Behavioral Changes:**
   - **Apathy and Depression:** Reduced motivation and interest in activities.
   - **Cognitive Impairment:** Problems with memory, attention, and executive function.

The progression of PSP is typically gradual but relentless, with symptoms worsening over time. Most individuals with PSP experience significant disability within a few years of onset, and the condition can eventually lead to severe physical and cognitive impairment.

Diagnosis and Medical Tests

Diagnosing PSP can be challenging due to its similarities with other neurological disorders. A thorough clinical evaluation is essential, often involving the following steps:

1. **Medical History and Symptom Review:** Detailed discussion of symptoms, medical history, and family history.
2. **Neurological Examination:** Assessment of motor functions, eye movements, speech, and cognitive abilities.
3. **Imaging Studies:** MRI or CT scans to rule out other conditions and identify characteristic brain changes associated with PSP.
4. **Specialized Tests:** PET or SPECT scans may be used in research settings to study brain function and tau protein distribution.

Early and accurate diagnosis is crucial for effective management and care planning. If you or a loved one is experiencing symptoms of PSP, it is essential to seek evaluation from a neurologist or specialist experienced in movement disorders.

Differentiating PSP from Other Neurodegenerative Disorders

PSP shares symptoms with several other neurodegenerative conditions, making differentiation critical for appropriate management. Key distinguishing features include:

- **Parkinson's Disease:** While both PSP and Parkinson's disease involve movement problems, PSP typically includes more severe postural instability and falls, as well as the characteristic eye movement abnormalities not seen in Parkinson's.
- **Corticobasal Degeneration (CBD):** Both PSP and CBD involve tau pathology, but CBD often presents with asymmetric motor symptoms and unique signs like alien limb phenomenon.

- **Multiple System Atrophy (MSA):** MSA involves autonomic dysfunction (e.g., blood pressure regulation issues) and lacks the specific eye movement abnormalities seen in PSP.

Accurate diagnosis requires careful evaluation by experienced healthcare professionals, often involving neurologists, neuropsychologists, and other specialists in movement disorders.

Conclusion

Understanding the basics of PSP, its causes, symptoms, and diagnostic process, is the first step in managing the condition effectively. This chapter has provided an overview of PSP, setting the stage for more detailed discussions on symptom management, practical tips, and support strategies in the following chapters. With the right knowledge and resources, individuals with PSP and their caregivers can navigate the challenges of this condition and improve their quality of life.

Chapter 2: Motor Symptom Management

Motor symptoms are among the most challenging aspects of Progressive Supranuclear Palsy (PSP). Managing these symptoms effectively can significantly improve quality of life for individuals with PSP and ease the caregiving process. This chapter will cover strategies and therapies to help manage bradykinesia, rigidity, balance issues, and more.

Strategies for Managing Bradykinesia and Rigidity

Bradykinesia, or the slowness of movement, and rigidity, or muscle stiffness, are hallmark symptoms of PSP. These symptoms can make everyday activities challenging. Here are some strategies to manage them:

1. **Regular Exercise:**
   - **Aerobic Exercise:** Activities like walking, swimming, or stationary biking can help maintain overall fitness and mobility.
   - **Strength Training:** Light weightlifting or resistance band exercises can help maintain muscle strength.
   - **Flexibility Exercises:** Stretching routines, such as yoga or Pilates, can help reduce muscle stiffness and improve flexibility.
2. **Physical Therapy:**
   - **Customized Exercise Programs:** A physical therapist can design a personalized exercise regimen tailored to the individual's abilities and needs.
   - **Balance and Gait Training:** Techniques to improve walking patterns and prevent falls.
   - **Manual Therapy:** Hands-on techniques to reduce muscle tension and improve mobility.

3. **Medications:**
    - **Levodopa:** Though not always effective in PSP, some individuals may benefit from this Parkinson's medication.
    - **Muscle Relaxants:** Medications like baclofen or tizanidine can help reduce muscle stiffness.
4. **Assistive Devices:**
    - **Canes or Walkers:** Providing additional support to improve balance and reduce the risk of falls.
    - **Wheelchairs:** For those with severe mobility issues, a wheelchair can provide independence and safety.

Tips for Improving Balance and Preventing Falls

Falls are a common and serious concern for individuals with PSP due to postural instability. Implementing the following tips can help reduce the risk of falls:

1. **Home Modifications:**
    - **Remove Clutter:** Keep floors clear of obstacles and clutter to prevent tripping.
    - **Install Handrails:** Add handrails in hallways, bathrooms, and stairways.
    - **Use Non-Slip Mats:** Place non-slip mats in the bathroom and other areas prone to wet floors.
2. **Balance Exercises:**
    - **Tai Chi:** This gentle martial art focuses on slow, controlled movements and can improve balance and coordination.
    - **Standing Balance Exercises:** Practice standing on one foot or shifting weight from one foot to the other while holding onto a sturdy support.
3. **Footwear:**
    - **Supportive Shoes:** Wear shoes with good arch support and non-slip soles.
    - **Avoid Loose Slippers:** Loose-fitting slippers can increase the risk of tripping.

4. **Caution with Movement:**
    - o **Move Slowly:** Encourage slow, deliberate movements when changing positions.
    - o **Use Mobility Aids:** Ensure the individual consistently uses canes, walkers, or other assistive devices.

Exercises and Physical Therapy

Regular exercise and physical therapy are crucial for managing motor symptoms in PSP. Here are some specific exercises and therapies that can be beneficial:

1. **Strengthening Exercises:**
    - o **Leg Lifts:** Strengthen leg muscles by lifting each leg while sitting or lying down.
    - o **Arm Raises:** Raise arms to the side or front to strengthen shoulder muscles.
2. **Flexibility Exercises:**
    - o **Hamstring Stretches:** Stretch the back of the thigh to improve leg flexibility.
    - o **Shoulder Stretches:** Stretch the shoulders and upper back to maintain upper body flexibility.
3. **Balance Exercises:**
    - o **Heel-to-Toe Walk:** Walk in a straight line, placing the heel of one foot directly in front of the toes of the other.
    - o **Standing on One Foot:** Practice standing on one foot for a few seconds at a time, using support if necessary.
4. **Physical Therapy Techniques:**
    - o **Gait Training:** Practice walking with proper form and rhythm to improve gait.
    - o **Postural Training:** Exercises to improve posture and prevent forward stooping.

Using Mobility Aids

Mobility aids can provide significant support for individuals with PSP, helping them maintain independence and reduce the risk of falls. Here are some commonly used aids:

1. **Canes:**
   - **Single-Point Canes:** Provide basic support for those with mild balance issues.
   - **Quad Canes:** Offer more stability with a wider base.
2. **Walkers:**
   - **Standard Walkers:** Provide stable support but require lifting to move.
   - **Rollators:** Walkers with wheels and a seat, allowing for easier movement and rest breaks.
3. **Wheelchairs:**
   - **Manual Wheelchairs:** Suitable for those who can still use their arms to propel themselves.
   - **Power Wheelchairs:** Offer independence for those with limited upper body strength.
4. **Other Aids:**
   - **Lift Chairs:** Assist in standing up from a seated position.
   - **Grab Bars:** Installed in key areas like bathrooms to provide support.

Conclusion

Managing motor symptoms in PSP is a multifaceted approach involving regular exercise, physical therapy, appropriate medications, and the use of assistive devices. By implementing these strategies, individuals with PSP can maintain their mobility and independence for as long as possible, while caregivers can provide more effective support. The next chapter will focus on managing eye movement and vision issues, another critical aspect of living with PSP.

Chapter 3: Eye Movement and Vision Issues

One of the defining characteristics of Progressive Supranuclear Palsy (PSP) is the difficulty with eye movements, particularly the inability to move the eyes up and down. These vision issues can significantly impact daily life, making tasks such as reading, navigating, and even social interactions challenging. This chapter will explore the common eye movement problems associated with PSP and provide practical strategies for managing these issues.

Understanding Eye Movement Problems in PSP

The eye movement difficulties in PSP, known as supranuclear gaze palsy, primarily affect vertical gaze (up and down movements). These problems occur because of the degeneration of specific brain areas that control eye movements. The key issues include:

1. **Supranuclear Gaze Palsy:** Difficulty moving the eyes up and down, while side-to-side movements may also be affected as the disease progresses.
2. **Blurred Vision:** Resulting from the inability to coordinate eye movements properly.
3. **Double Vision (Diplopia):** Caused by misalignment of the eyes, leading to seeing two images instead of one.
4. **Difficulty with Convergence:** Trouble focusing on objects that are close, making reading and other close-up tasks challenging.

Managing Blurred Vision and Double Vision

1. **Prism Glasses:**
    - **Purpose:** Prism glasses can help correct double vision by aligning the images seen by each eye.
    - **Consultation:** An optometrist or ophthalmologist can prescribe prism glasses tailored to the individual's needs.

2. **Visual Aids:**
    - o **Magnifying Glasses:** Useful for reading and other close-up tasks.
    - o **Large Print Materials:** Books, labels, and other materials in large print can reduce eye strain.
3. **Environmental Adjustments:**
    - o **Good Lighting:** Ensure well-lit environments to reduce the strain on the eyes.
    - o **High-Contrast Colors:** Use high-contrast colors for important objects and text to make them easier to see.

Tips for Adapting to Vision Changes

1. **Home Modifications:**
    - o **Clear Pathways:** Remove tripping hazards and ensure clear, unobstructed pathways.
    - o **Use of Contrasting Colors:** Highlight edges of steps, doorframes, and other potential hazards with contrasting colors.
2. **Daily Living Aids:**
    - o **Voice-Activated Devices:** Use smart home devices that respond to voice commands to reduce the need for visual tasks.
    - o **Tactile Markings:** Place tactile markers on frequently used items such as remote controls and appliances.
3. **Reading and Writing:**
    - o **Audiobooks and E-Books:** These can be alternatives to traditional reading, allowing users to listen instead of read.
    - o **Voice-to-Text Technology:** Use software that converts spoken words into text, reducing the need for writing.

Role of Eye Exercises and Therapies

Although PSP cannot be cured, certain exercises and therapies can help manage eye movement issues and improve functional vision:

1. **Eye Movement Exercises:**
    - **Tracking Exercises:** Practice following a moving object with the eyes to improve coordination.
    - **Focus Shifting:** Move focus from near to far objects to enhance flexibility in eye movement.
2. **Occupational Therapy:**
    - **Visual Motor Training:** Occupational therapists can provide exercises to improve hand-eye coordination and visual motor skills.
    - **Adaptive Strategies:** Therapists can teach strategies to compensate for vision loss in daily activities.
3. **Consultation with Eye Specialists:**
    - **Regular Check-ups:** Regular visits to an ophthalmologist or neuro-ophthalmologist can help monitor and manage vision changes.
    - **Customized Interventions:** Specialists can provide tailored solutions and interventions based on the individual's specific vision issues.

Conclusion

Managing eye movement and vision issues in PSP requires a combination of practical adjustments, visual aids, exercises, and professional interventions. By implementing these strategies, individuals with PSP can better navigate their environment and maintain a higher quality of life. The next chapter will address speech and swallowing difficulties, another significant aspect of living with PSP.

Chapter 4: Speech and Swallowing Difficulties

Speech and swallowing difficulties are common and challenging symptoms of Progressive Supranuclear Palsy (PSP). These issues can significantly impact communication, nutrition, and overall quality of life. This chapter will explore common speech and swallowing problems associated with PSP and provide strategies and therapies to manage them effectively.

Common Speech and Swallowing Issues

1. **Dysarthria:**
   - **Symptoms:** Slurred or slow speech, making it difficult to communicate clearly.
   - **Causes:** Muscle weakness and impaired coordination of the muscles used in speech.
2. **Dysphagia:**
   - **Symptoms:** Difficulty swallowing, leading to choking, aspiration, and potential malnutrition.
   - **Causes:** Weakness and lack of coordination in the muscles involved in swallowing.
3. **Communication Challenges:**
   - **Reduced Vocal Volume:** Soft voice or whispering due to weak vocal cords.
   - **Monotone Speech:** Lack of inflection or variation in speech tone.

Techniques for Improving Speech Clarity

1. **Speech Therapy:**
   - **Articulation Exercises:** Practice specific sounds and words to improve clarity.
   - **Breathing Exercises:** Enhance breath control to support speech.
   - **Voice Amplification:** Use devices that amplify the voice to make communication easier.

2. **Assistive Communication Devices:**
    - ○ **Speech Generating Devices (SGDs):** Electronic devices that produce speech based on user input.
    - ○ **Communication Apps:** Applications on tablets and smartphones that assist with communication.
    - ○ **Picture Boards:** Use of visual aids and symbols to facilitate communication.
3. **Techniques for Caregivers and Family:**
    - ○ **Active Listening:** Pay close attention and be patient, allowing extra time for the person to speak.
    - ○ **Use of Gestures:** Encourage the use of gestures and non-verbal communication.
    - ○ **Repeat and Confirm:** Repeat back what you have understood to ensure clarity.

Strategies for Safe Swallowing

1. **Swallowing Techniques:**
    - ○ **Chin Tuck:** Tucking the chin down while swallowing to prevent food from entering the airway.
    - ○ **Small Bites and Sips:** Taking smaller amounts of food and liquid to reduce choking risk.
    - ○ **Double Swallowing:** Swallowing twice to ensure food is completely cleared from the throat.
2. **Diet Modifications:**
    - ○ **Thickened Liquids:** Use thickening agents to make liquids easier to swallow.
    - ○ **Soft Foods:** Incorporate soft and easy-to-swallow foods into the diet.
    - ○ **Avoid Dry and Crumbly Foods:** These can be difficult to swallow and increase choking risk.
3. **Feeding Techniques:**
    - ○ **Upright Positioning:** Ensure the individual is sitting upright during meals to aid swallowing.
    - ○ **Slow Eating Pace:** Encourage slow eating to allow adequate time for safe swallowing.
    - ○ **Monitor During Meals:** Caregivers should closely monitor for signs of choking or difficulty.

Speech and Language Therapy

1. **Role of Speech-Language Pathologists (SLPs):**
   - **Assessment and Diagnosis:** SLPs assess speech and swallowing functions to identify specific challenges.
   - **Personalized Treatment Plans:** Develop individualized therapy plans to address the unique needs of each person.
   - **Therapeutic Exercises:** Provide exercises to strengthen the muscles involved in speech and swallowing.
2. **Therapeutic Techniques:**
   - **Lee Silverman Voice Treatment (LSVT LOUD):** An intensive therapy focusing on increasing vocal loudness.
   - **Swallowing Therapy:** Exercises and techniques to improve swallowing safety and efficiency.
   - **Communication Strategies:** Training in alternative communication methods and tools.
3. **Support and Education:**
   - **Caregiver Training:** Educate caregivers on how to assist with speech and swallowing exercises.
   - **Ongoing Monitoring:** Regular follow-ups to adjust therapy plans as needed.

Conclusion

Managing speech and swallowing difficulties in PSP requires a multidisciplinary approach involving speech therapy, assistive devices, dietary modifications, and caregiver support. By implementing these strategies, individuals with PSP can improve their communication and maintain better nutrition and safety while eating. The next chapter will address cognitive and behavioral changes, providing strategies to manage these symptoms effectively.

Chapter 5: Cognitive and Behavioral Changes

Progressive Supranuclear Palsy (PSP) not only affects motor functions and speech but also leads to significant cognitive and behavioral changes. These changes can be particularly challenging for both individuals with PSP and their caregivers. This chapter will explore the common cognitive and behavioral symptoms associated with PSP and offer strategies to manage them effectively.

Identifying Cognitive Symptoms

Cognitive changes in PSP can vary but commonly include:

1. **Memory Impairment:**
   - Difficulty recalling recent events or information.
   - Challenges with short-term memory.
2. **Executive Dysfunction:**
   - Problems with planning, organizing, and completing tasks.
   - Difficulty in making decisions and problem-solving.
3. **Attention and Concentration:**
   - Reduced ability to focus on tasks.
   - Easily distracted and difficulty maintaining attention.
4. **Language Difficulties:**
   - Problems finding the right words.
   - Difficulty understanding complex sentences.

Strategies for Managing Behavioral Changes

Behavioral changes can be distressing for both the person with PSP and their caregivers. Common behavioral symptoms include apathy, depression, irritability, and impulsivity. Here are some strategies to manage these changes:

1. **Establish Routines:**
    o Consistent daily routines can help reduce confusion and anxiety.
    o Structured schedules for meals, activities, and rest periods.
2. **Create a Supportive Environment:**
    o Simplify the environment by reducing clutter and minimizing distractions.
    o Ensure a calm and safe space for the person with PSP.
3. **Behavioral Interventions:**
    o **Positive Reinforcement:** Encourage and reward positive behaviors.
    o **Redirecting Attention:** Gently redirect inappropriate behaviors or comments without confrontation.
4. **Professional Support:**
    o **Counseling and Therapy:** Access to mental health professionals for both the person with PSP and their caregivers.
    o **Support Groups:** Joining support groups can provide emotional support and practical advice.

Cognitive Stimulation Activities

Engaging in cognitive activities can help maintain mental function and provide a sense of accomplishment. Here are some recommended activities:

1. **Puzzles and Games:**
    o Activities like crosswords, Sudoku, and jigsaw puzzles can stimulate cognitive function.
    o Board games that require strategic thinking and memory.
2. **Reading and Writing:**
    o Reading books, newspapers, or magazines to maintain language skills.

o Writing letters, keeping a journal, or engaging in creative writing.
3. **Arts and Crafts:**
   o Drawing, painting, knitting, or other craft activities that engage the mind and hands.
4. **Music and Singing:**
   o Listening to music, singing, or playing a musical instrument can be both stimulating and soothing.

Support for Emotional Well-being

Emotional well-being is crucial for individuals with PSP and their caregivers. Here are some strategies to support emotional health:

1. **Counseling and Therapy:**
   o **Individual Therapy:** Professional counseling to address depression, anxiety, and other emotional challenges.
   o **Family Therapy:** Therapy sessions involving family members to improve communication and support.
2. **Mindfulness and Relaxation Techniques:**
   o **Meditation:** Practicing mindfulness meditation to reduce stress and improve emotional regulation.
   o **Relaxation Exercises:** Techniques such as deep breathing, progressive muscle relaxation, and guided imagery.
3. **Social Engagement:**
   o **Maintaining Social Connections:** Encourage visits with family and friends, participation in social activities, and community involvement.
   o **Support Groups:** Joining groups for individuals with PSP and their caregivers can provide mutual support and understanding.
4. **Physical Activity:**
   o Regular physical exercise, such as walking, swimming, or yoga, can boost mood and reduce anxiety.

Conclusion

Managing cognitive and behavioral changes in PSP requires a comprehensive approach that includes establishing routines, creating a supportive environment, engaging in cognitive activities, and seeking professional support. By implementing these strategies, individuals with PSP and their caregivers can better cope with these challenging symptoms and improve their quality of life. The next chapter will address managing pain and discomfort, another critical aspect of living with PSP.

Chapter 6: Managing Pain and Discomfort

Pain and discomfort are common and distressing symptoms for individuals with Progressive Supranuclear Palsy (PSP). Effective management of these symptoms is essential to improving the quality of life for both individuals with PSP and their caregivers. This chapter will explore the sources of pain in PSP and provide strategies for pain relief and comfort.

Understanding Sources of Pain in PSP

Pain in PSP can arise from various sources, including:

1. **Muscle Rigidity and Spasticity:**
    - Continuous muscle tension leading to discomfort and pain.
    - Often affects the neck, back, and limbs.
2. **Joint Pain:**
    - Stiff joints due to lack of movement and muscle rigidity.
    - Can result from abnormal postures and limited mobility.
3. **Neuropathic Pain:**
    - Pain resulting from nerve damage or dysfunction.
    - Often described as burning, tingling, or shooting pain.
4. **Secondary Conditions:**
    - Pain associated with pressure sores, constipation, or urinary tract infections.

Pain Relief Strategies

1. **Medications:**
    - **Muscle Relaxants:** Medications like baclofen or tizanidine can help reduce muscle stiffness and spasticity.

- o **Analgesics:** Over-the-counter pain relievers such as acetaminophen or ibuprofen can manage mild to moderate pain.
  - o **Prescription Pain Medications:** For severe pain, stronger medications may be prescribed by a healthcare professional.
2. **Physical Therapy:**
  - o **Stretching and Strengthening Exercises:** Regular exercises to maintain flexibility and muscle strength.
  - o **Massage Therapy:** Professional massages to relieve muscle tension and improve circulation.
  - o **Hydrotherapy:** Water-based exercises can provide gentle resistance and support movement.
3. **Complementary Therapies:**
  - o **Acupuncture:** May help alleviate pain and improve overall well-being.
  - o **Heat and Cold Therapy:** Applying heat packs or cold compresses to painful areas can reduce pain and inflammation.
  - o **Transcutaneous Electrical Nerve Stimulation (TENS):** A device that delivers electrical impulses to reduce pain perception.

Managing Discomfort

1. **Positioning and Mobility:**
  - o **Frequent Position Changes:** Regularly changing positions to prevent pressure sores and improve comfort.
  - o **Supportive Cushions and Mattresses:** Using specialized cushions and mattresses to provide better support and reduce discomfort.
2. **Assistive Devices:**
  - o **Adjustable Beds:** Beds that can be adjusted to different positions to enhance comfort.
  - o **Wheelchairs and Recliners:** Providing proper seating support to reduce pain and discomfort during daily activities.

3. **Daily Living Adjustments:**
   - ○ **Adaptive Clothing:** Wearing loose-fitting and easy-to-remove clothing to reduce discomfort.
   - ○ **Assistive Eating Utensils:** Using special utensils designed for individuals with limited hand function to make eating easier.

Complementary Therapies

1. **Mind-Body Techniques:**
   - ○ **Meditation and Relaxation Exercises:** Practicing mindfulness and relaxation techniques to manage pain and stress.
   - ○ **Breathing Exercises:** Deep breathing exercises to promote relaxation and reduce pain perception.
2. **Aromatherapy:**
   - ○ **Essential Oils:** Using oils such as lavender or chamomile in diffusers or as massage oils to promote relaxation and alleviate pain.
3. **Music Therapy:**
   - ○ **Listening to Soothing Music:** Can help distract from pain and promote relaxation.

Medications for Pain Management

1. **Non-Opioid Pain Relievers:**
   - ○ **Acetaminophen:** Effective for mild to moderate pain without the risk of addiction.
   - ○ **NSAIDs:** Non-steroidal anti-inflammatory drugs like ibuprofen can reduce inflammation and pain.
2. **Opioid Pain Relievers:**
   - ○ **For Severe Pain:** Prescribed for short-term use in severe pain cases, with careful monitoring due to the risk of dependency and side effects.
3. **Topical Analgesics:**
   - ○ **Creams and Gels:** Applied directly to the skin over painful areas to provide localized relief.

Conclusion

Effective pain and discomfort management in PSP involves a combination of medications, physical therapy, complementary therapies, and lifestyle adjustments. By implementing these strategies, individuals with PSP can experience significant relief, leading to improved comfort and quality of life. The next chapter will address daily living and practical tips, providing guidance on adapting the home environment, establishing routines, and using assistive devices to enhance daily activities.

Chapter 7: Daily Living and Practical Tips

Adapting daily routines and the living environment can significantly improve the quality of life for individuals with Progressive Supranuclear Palsy (PSP) and their caregivers. This chapter provides practical tips for managing daily activities, making home modifications, and using assistive devices to maintain independence and safety.

Adapting the Home Environment

Creating a safe and accessible living space is crucial for individuals with PSP. Here are some recommendations:

1. **Safety Modifications:**
   - **Remove Clutter:** Keep floors clear of obstacles to prevent tripping and falls.
   - **Install Grab Bars:** Place grab bars in the bathroom, near the toilet, and in the shower for added support.
   - **Use Non-Slip Mats:** In the bathroom and kitchen, use non-slip mats to reduce the risk of slipping.
2. **Mobility Aids:**
   - **Ramps:** Install ramps for easy access to different levels of the house.
   - **Handrails:** Ensure that stairs and hallways have sturdy handrails.
3. **Lighting:**
   - **Bright Lighting:** Ensure that all areas of the home are well-lit to improve visibility.
   - **Night Lights:** Place night lights in the bedroom, hallways, and bathroom to help with nighttime navigation.

Daily Routines and Activities

Establishing consistent daily routines can help manage PSP symptoms and reduce stress for both individuals with PSP and their caregivers.

1. **Structured Schedule:**
   - **Set a Routine:** Create a daily schedule that includes regular times for meals, exercise, rest, and activities.
   - **Consistency:** Stick to the routine as much as possible to provide a sense of stability and predictability.
2. **Activity Planning:**
   - **Balance Activity and Rest:** Plan activities to avoid fatigue. Include rest periods throughout the day.
   - **Engage in Enjoyable Activities:** Continue to engage in hobbies and activities that the individual enjoys and can safely perform.
3. **Task Simplification:**
   - **Break Tasks into Steps:** Simplify complex tasks by breaking them down into smaller, manageable steps.
   - **Use Visual Aids:** Create checklists or visual schedules to help with task completion.

Communication Strategies

Effective communication is vital for maintaining relationships and ensuring that needs are met. Here are some tips:

1. **Clear Speech:**
   - **Speak Slowly and Clearly:** Ensure that speech is slow and clear to improve understanding.
   - **Use Short Sentences:** Keep sentences short and simple.

2. **Non-Verbal Communication:**
    - o **Gestures:** Use gestures and facial expressions to support verbal communication.
    - o **Writing:** Use writing or drawing to convey messages when speech is difficult.
3. **Assistive Technology:**
    - o **Communication Devices:** Utilize communication devices or apps designed to assist with speech difficulties.

Mobility Aids and Assistive Devices

Using the right mobility aids and assistive devices can enhance independence and safety.

1. **Walking Aids:**
    - o **Canes and Walkers:** Provide stability and support while walking.
    - o **Rollators:** Walkers with wheels and a seat for resting.
2. **Wheelchairs and Scooters:**
    - o **Manual Wheelchairs:** For those who need support but can still propel themselves.
    - o **Electric Scooters:** Provide mobility for longer distances or those with limited strength.
3. **Adaptive Equipment:**
    - o **Reachers and Grabbers:** Help retrieve objects without bending or stretching.
    - o **Adaptive Utensils:** Specially designed utensils to aid with eating and drinking.

Nutrition and Diet

Maintaining a healthy diet is essential for overall well-being and managing PSP symptoms.

1. **Balanced Diet:**
    o   **Nutrient-Rich Foods:** Include a variety of fruits, vegetables, whole grains, lean proteins, and healthy fats.
    o   **Hydration:** Ensure adequate fluid intake to prevent dehydration.
2. **Meal Preparation:**
    o   **Easy-to-Chew Foods:** Prepare meals with soft, easy-to-chew foods to accommodate swallowing difficulties.
    o   **Small, Frequent Meals:** Eating smaller, more frequent meals can help manage appetite and nutrition.
3. **Dietary Modifications:**
    o   **Thickened Liquids:** Use thickening agents for liquids to reduce the risk of aspiration.
    o   **High-Calorie Foods:** Include high-calorie foods if weight loss is a concern.

Conclusion

Adapting the home environment, establishing daily routines, and using assistive devices are crucial steps in managing daily life with PSP. These practical tips can help individuals with PSP maintain their independence and improve their quality of life. The next chapter will focus on nutrition and diet, offering detailed advice on dietary adjustments and meal planning to support health and well-being in PSP.

Chapter 8: Nutrition and Diet

Maintaining a proper diet and nutrition is essential for individuals with Progressive Supranuclear Palsy (PSP) to ensure overall health, manage symptoms, and improve quality of life. This chapter provides guidance on dietary recommendations, managing weight and nutritional intake, and meal planning to address the specific needs of individuals with PSP.

Importance of Nutrition in PSP

Proper nutrition plays a crucial role in managing PSP by:

- Supporting overall health and energy levels.
- Helping to maintain a healthy weight.
- Managing swallowing difficulties.
- Reducing the risk of complications like aspiration pneumonia.

Dietary Recommendations

1. **Balanced Diet:**
   - **Fruits and Vegetables:** Aim to include a variety of colorful fruits and vegetables in every meal for essential vitamins and minerals.
   - **Whole Grains:** Choose whole grains such as brown rice, quinoa, and whole wheat bread for added fiber and nutrients.
   - **Lean Proteins:** Include lean protein sources like chicken, fish, beans, and legumes to support muscle maintenance.
   - **Healthy Fats:** Incorporate healthy fats from sources such as avocados, nuts, seeds, and olive oil.
2. **Hydration:**
   - **Adequate Fluid Intake:** Ensure regular intake of fluids to stay hydrated. Water, herbal teas, and clear broths are good options.

- o **Monitor for Dehydration:** Watch for signs of dehydration such as dark urine, dry mouth, and fatigue.

Managing Weight and Nutritional Intake

1. **Maintaining a Healthy Weight:**
   - o **Regular Monitoring:** Regularly check weight to monitor for unintentional weight loss or gain.
   - o **Nutrient-Dense Foods:** Choose nutrient-dense foods that provide essential nutrients without excessive calories.
2. **Addressing Swallowing Difficulties:**
   - o **Texture Modifications:** Modify food textures to make swallowing easier. Use pureed, minced, or soft foods as needed.
   - o **Thickened Liquids:** Use commercially available thickening agents to make liquids easier to swallow and reduce the risk of aspiration.
3. **Small, Frequent Meals:**
   - o **Meal Frequency:** Eating smaller, more frequent meals can help manage appetite and ensure adequate nutrition.
   - o **Caloric Intake:** Include high-calorie, nutrient-dense snacks such as smoothies, yogurt, and nut butter to increase calorie intake.

Meal Planning and Preparation Tips

1. **Meal Planning:**
   - o **Weekly Planning:** Plan meals and snacks for the week to ensure a balanced and varied diet.
   - o **Incorporate Favorites:** Include favorite foods to encourage appetite and enjoyment of meals.
2. **Easy-to-Prepare Meals:**
   - o **Simple Recipes:** Choose recipes that are easy to prepare and require minimal cooking time.

  o **Batch Cooking:** Prepare larger quantities of food and freeze individual portions for quick and easy meals.

3. **Adaptive Cooking Tools:**
  o **Ergonomic Utensils:** Use ergonomic utensils and kitchen tools designed for individuals with limited hand function.
  o **Blenders and Food Processors:** These can be useful for preparing pureed and soft foods.

Nutritional Supplements

1. **Multivitamins:**
  o **Supplementation:** Consider a daily multivitamin to ensure adequate intake of essential vitamins and minerals, especially if dietary intake is limited.
2. **Protein Supplements:**
  o **Protein Shakes:** Use protein shakes or powders to increase protein intake if consuming enough through diet is challenging.
3. **Consultation with a Dietitian:**
  o **Professional Guidance:** A registered dietitian can provide personalized nutritional advice and create tailored meal plans to meet specific needs.

Monitoring and Adjusting Diet

1. **Regular Assessment:**
  o **Nutritional Assessments:** Regularly assess nutritional status with healthcare professionals to ensure dietary needs are being met.
  o **Adjustments:** Make dietary adjustments as needed based on changes in health status and nutritional needs.
2. **Swallowing Evaluations:**
  o **Speech-Language Pathologists:** Work with SLP for regular swallowing evaluations to adjust food textures and liquid consistencies as needed.

Conclusion

Proper nutrition and diet management are critical components of care for individuals with PSP. By following these dietary recommendations, managing weight and nutritional intake, and planning meals effectively, individuals with PSP can improve their overall health and quality of life. The next chapter will focus on emotional and psychological support, providing strategies for coping with the emotional challenges of living with PSP.

Chapter 9: Emotional and Psychological Support

Living with Progressive Supranuclear Palsy (PSP) can be emotionally and psychologically challenging for both individuals with the condition and their caregivers. Addressing these challenges is crucial for maintaining overall well-being and quality of life. This chapter provides strategies for coping with the emotional impact of PSP, managing stress and anxiety, and seeking support for both patients and caregivers.

Coping with the Diagnosis

1. **Understanding the Condition:**
   - o **Educate Yourself:** Learn as much as possible about PSP to understand its progression and what to expect.
   - o **Set Realistic Expectations:** Recognize the challenges ahead and set achievable goals.
2. **Accepting Emotions:**
   - o **Acknowledge Feelings:** Allow yourself to feel a range of emotions, including sadness, anger, and frustration.
   - o **Seek Support:** Talk to friends, family, or a therapist about your feelings.
3. **Finding Meaning:**
   - o **Focus on What Matters:** Identify activities and relationships that bring joy and purpose.
   - o **Adapt Activities:** Modify favorite activities to make them accessible and enjoyable.

Managing Stress and Anxiety

1. **Stress-Reduction Techniques:**
   - o **Mindfulness Meditation:** Practice mindfulness and meditation to stay present and reduce stress.

- o **Deep Breathing Exercises:** Use deep breathing techniques to calm the mind and body.
2. **Physical Activity:**
   - o **Regular Exercise:** Engage in regular physical activity, such as walking or yoga, to reduce stress and improve mood.
   - o **Gentle Movements:** Even light stretching or seated exercises can be beneficial.
3. **Healthy Lifestyle:**
   - o **Balanced Diet:** Maintain a healthy diet to support physical and emotional well-being.
   - o **Adequate Sleep:** Ensure sufficient sleep to help manage stress and anxiety.

Support for Caregivers

1. **Self-Care:**
   - o **Take Breaks:** Regularly take time for yourself to rest and recharge.
   - o **Healthy Habits:** Maintain your own health through balanced nutrition, exercise, and sleep.
2. **Seek Help:**
   - o **Ask for Assistance:** Don't hesitate to ask family, friends, or professional caregivers for help.
   - o **Respite Care:** Consider respite care services to give yourself a break from caregiving duties.
3. **Emotional Support:**
   - o **Support Groups:** Join support groups for caregivers to share experiences and gain support.
   - o **Therapy:** Seek counseling or therapy to manage the emotional challenges of caregiving.

Counseling and Support Groups

1. **Individual Therapy:**
   - o **Professional Help:** Work with a therapist to address personal emotional and psychological challenges.

- o **Cognitive Behavioral Therapy (CBT):** CBT can help manage negative thoughts and develop coping strategies.
2. **Family Therapy:**
   - o **Family Dynamics:** Address family dynamics and improve communication and support within the family.
   - o **Shared Understanding:** Help family members understand PSP and its impact on everyone involved.
3. **Support Groups:**
   - o **Peer Support:** Join support groups for individuals with PSP and their caregivers to share experiences and gain mutual support.
   - o **Online Communities:** Participate in online forums and social media groups for additional support and information.

Mindfulness and Relaxation Techniques

1. **Mindfulness Practices:**
   - o **Meditation:** Regular meditation practice can help reduce stress and improve emotional well-being.
   - o **Mindful Breathing:** Focus on your breath to bring awareness and calm to the present moment.
2. **Relaxation Techniques:**
   - o **Progressive Muscle Relaxation:** Gradually tense and then relax each muscle group to reduce physical tension.
   - o **Guided Imagery:** Use visualization techniques to imagine calming and peaceful scenes.
3. **Creative Outlets:**
   - o **Art Therapy:** Engage in creative activities like drawing, painting, or crafting to express emotions.
   - o **Music Therapy:** Listening to or playing music can be soothing and emotionally uplifting.

Conclusion

Emotional and psychological support is a vital aspect of managing PSP for both individuals with the condition and their caregivers. By implementing these strategies for coping with the diagnosis, managing stress and anxiety, and seeking support, individuals and caregivers can improve their emotional well-being and overall quality of life. The next chapter will address advanced care planning, providing guidance on legal and financial considerations, planning for future care needs, and exploring hospice and palliative care options.

Chapter 10: Advanced Care Planning

Planning for the future is an essential aspect of managing Progressive Supranuclear Palsy (PSP). Advanced care planning helps individuals with PSP and their families make informed decisions about legal, financial, and medical matters. This chapter will provide guidance on legal and financial planning, preparing for future care needs, and exploring hospice and palliative care options.

Legal and Financial Considerations

1. **Establishing Legal Documents:**
   - **Durable Power of Attorney:** Designate someone to make financial and legal decisions on your behalf.
   - **Medical Power of Attorney:** Appoint a trusted person to make healthcare decisions if you are unable to do so.
   - **Living Will:** Outline your preferences for medical treatments and interventions in case you are unable to communicate your wishes.
2. **Estate Planning:**
   - **Will and Testament:** Ensure you have a will that specifies how your assets will be distributed after your death.
   - **Trusts:** Consider setting up a trust to manage your assets and provide for your family's future needs.
3. **Financial Planning:**
   - **Budgeting for Care:** Plan for the costs associated with PSP care, including medications, therapies, and caregiving services.
   - **Insurance:** Review your health, disability, and long-term care insurance policies to ensure adequate coverage.

- o **Government Benefits:** Explore eligibility for government programs such as Social Security Disability Insurance (SSDI) and Medicaid.

Planning for Future Care Needs

1. **Assessing Care Needs:**
   - o **Current and Future Needs:** Evaluate your current care needs and anticipate future changes as PSP progresses.
   - o **Caregiving Arrangements:** Determine whether care will be provided at home, by family members, or through professional caregivers.
2. **Home Care Planning:**
   - o **Home Modifications:** Make necessary modifications to your home to ensure safety and accessibility.
   - o **Hiring Caregivers:** Consider hiring professional caregivers to provide assistance with daily activities and medical care.
3. **Residential Care Options:**
   - o **Assisted Living Facilities:** Explore assisted living facilities that offer support with daily activities while promoting independence.
   - o **Nursing Homes:** Consider nursing homes for individuals who require more intensive medical care and supervision.

Hospice and Palliative Care

1. **Understanding Hospice Care:**
   - o **Hospice Philosophy:** Hospice care focuses on providing comfort and quality of life for individuals with terminal illnesses.
   - o **Eligibility:** Hospice care is typically available to individuals with a prognosis of six months or less to live.

2. **Palliative Care:**
    - **Comprehensive Support:** Palliative care provides relief from symptoms and stress associated with serious illnesses, regardless of the prognosis.
    - **Interdisciplinary Approach:** Palliative care teams include doctors, nurses, social workers, and chaplains who work together to address physical, emotional, and spiritual needs.
3. **End-of-Life Planning:**
    - **Advance Directives:** Ensure that your advance directives are up-to-date and reflect your current wishes.
    - **Discussing Wishes:** Have open and honest conversations with your family and healthcare providers about your end-of-life preferences.
    - **Comfort Measures:** Focus on comfort measures that prioritize pain management and quality of life.

Conclusion

Advanced care planning is a critical component of managing PSP, allowing individuals and their families to make informed decisions about legal, financial, and medical matters. By establishing legal documents, planning for future care needs, and exploring hospice and palliative care options, individuals with PSP can ensure their wishes are respected and their needs are met. The next chapter will address resources and support, providing information on finding medical experts, support organizations, and online communities to assist individuals with PSP and their caregivers.

Chapter 11: Resources and Support

Navigating Progressive Supranuclear Palsy (PSP) can be overwhelming, but numerous resources and support systems are available to help individuals with PSP and their caregivers. This chapter provides information on finding medical experts, support organizations, online communities, and additional resources to enhance the support network for those affected by PSP.

Finding Medical Experts and Specialists

1. **Neurologists:**
   - **Movement Disorder Specialists:** Seek out neurologists who specialize in movement disorders, as they have specific expertise in managing PSP.
   - **Comprehensive Care Centers:** Consider visiting comprehensive care centers that offer multidisciplinary teams of specialists.
2. **Physical and Occupational Therapists:**
   - **Customized Therapy Plans:** Work with therapists to develop personalized exercise and rehabilitation programs.
   - **Assistive Devices:** Therapists can recommend and train individuals to use assistive devices to improve mobility and independence.
3. **Speech-Language Pathologists:**
   - **Speech and Swallowing Therapy:** Engage with speech-language pathologists to address communication and swallowing difficulties.
   - **Alternative Communication:** Explore alternative communication methods and devices.
4. **Palliative Care Specialists:**
   - **Symptom Management:** Palliative care teams can help manage symptoms and improve quality of life.
   - **Holistic Support:** These specialists provide comprehensive support addressing physical, emotional, and spiritual needs.

Support Organizations and Foundations

1. **PSP-Specific Organizations:**
    - **CCF for PSP Awareness:** Provides support groups, resources and respite for individuals and caregivers.
    - **CurePSP:** Offers resources, support, and information specifically for PSP, including educational materials, support groups, and research funding.
    - **PSP Association:** Provides support services, advocacy, and information for individuals with PSP and their families.
2. **Parkinson's Disease Organizations:**
    - **Parkinson's Foundation:** While focused on Parkinson's disease, this organization provides resources and support that can also benefit those with PSP.
    - **Michael J. Fox Foundation:** Offers information on research and clinical trials that may be relevant to PSP.
3. **Neurological Disorder Organizations:**
    - **National Institute of Neurological Disorders and Stroke (NINDS):** Provides comprehensive information on PSP and other neurological conditions.
    - **American Academy of Neurology (AAN):** Offers resources and directories to find neurologists and specialists.

Online Communities and Forums

1. **Support Groups:**
    - **Online Support Groups:** Join online support groups where individuals with PSP and caregivers can share experiences, advice, and encouragement.

- o **Social Media Groups:** Participate in social media communities focused on PSP for peer support and information sharing.
2. **Educational Webinars and Videos:**
   - o **Webinars:** Attend educational webinars hosted by PSP organizations to stay informed about the latest research and management strategies.
   - o **Instructional Videos:** Access instructional videos on exercises, assistive devices, and caregiving techniques.
3. **Blogs and Personal Stories:**
   - o **Patient and Caregiver Blogs:** Read blogs and personal stories from individuals living with PSP and their caregivers to gain insights and inspiration.
   - o **Forums and Discussion Boards:** Engage in forums and discussion boards to ask questions and receive support from the PSP community.

Recommended Reading and Websites

1. **Books on PSP:**
   - o **"The PSP Chronicles" by Tim Brown:** Practical advice and personal stories from Tim living with PSP.
2. **Educational Websites:**
   - o **CCF for PSP Awareness-** www.pspawareness.com
   - o **CurePSP-** www.curepsp.org
   - o **PSP Association-** www.pspassociation.org.uk
3. **Research and Clinical Trials:**
   - o **ClinicalTrials.gov:** Search for ongoing clinical trials related to PSP to learn about new treatments and research opportunities.
   - o **National Institutes of Health (NIH):** Access research updates and publications related to PSP.

Conclusion

Accessing resources and support is essential for managing PSP effectively. By connecting with medical experts, support organizations, online communities, and educational materials, individuals with PSP and their caregivers can build a strong support network and stay informed about the latest advancements in care and research.

Appendices

The appendices provide additional resources, tools, and information to support individuals with Progressive Supranuclear Palsy (PSP) and their caregivers. This section includes a glossary of terms, frequently asked questions, sample care plans, and contact information for support services.

Glossary of Terms

- **Bradykinesia:** Slowness of movement, often seen in neurodegenerative diseases like PSP.
- **Dysarthria:** Difficulty in articulating words due to problems with the muscles that produce speech.
- **Dysphagia:** Difficulty swallowing.
- **Neurodegenerative:** Refers to diseases characterized by the progressive degeneration of nerve cells.
- **Palliative Care:** Specialized medical care focused on providing relief from the symptoms and stress of a serious illness.
- **Supranuclear Gaze Palsy:** A condition where individuals have difficulty moving their eyes, particularly in the vertical direction.

Frequently Asked Questions

1. **What is Progressive Supranuclear Palsy (PSP)?**
   - PSP is a rare, progressive brain disorder that affects movement, balance, vision, speech, and swallowing.
2. **What are the early signs of PSP?**
   - Early signs include unsteady walking, unexplained falls, stiffness, and difficulty with eye movements.
3. **How is PSP diagnosed?**
   - PSP is diagnosed through a combination of clinical evaluations, neurological exams, and imaging tests like MRI.
4. **Is there a cure for PSP?**
   - There is currently no cure for PSP, but treatments are available to manage symptoms and improve quality of life.
5. **What types of treatments are available for PSP?**
   - Treatments include medications, physical therapy, speech therapy, and occupational therapy to manage symptoms.
6. **How can caregivers support someone with PSP?**
   - Caregivers can support by helping with daily activities, providing emotional support, and seeking professional help when needed.

Sample Care Plans and Checklists

Daily Care Plan:

Time	Activity	Notes
7:00 AM	Morning Medication	Ensure medications are taken as prescribed
8:00 AM	Breakfast	Prepare a nutritious, easy-to-eat meal
9:00 AM	Physical Therapy Exercises	Follow exercises recommended by the therapist
10:00 AM	Rest Period	Allow for a short rest or quiet time
11:00 AM	Leisure Activity	Engage in a favorite hobby or activity
12:00 PM	Lunch	Serve a balanced, easy-to-swallow meal
1:00 PM	Afternoon Medication	Administer medications as prescribed
2:00 PM	Social Interaction	Spend time with family or friends
3:00 PM	Rest Period	Allow for a nap or quiet time
4:00 PM	Light Exercise	Gentle stretching or walking
5:00 PM	Dinner	Prepare a nutritious, easy-to-eat meal
6:00 PM	Evening Medication	Ensure medications are taken as prescribed
7:00 PM	Leisure Activity	Engage in a relaxing activity
8:00 PM	Bedtime Routine	Assist with personal care and prepare for bed

Home Safety Checklist:

- Remove tripping hazards (e.g., loose rugs, clutter).
- Install grab bars in the bathroom.
- Ensure good lighting throughout the home.
- Use non-slip mats in the bathroom and kitchen.
- Keep frequently used items within easy reach.
- Check that mobility aids are in good condition.

Contact Information for Support Services

1. **CCF for PSP Awareness**
   - Website: www.pspawareness.com
   - Phone: 905-616-9433
   - Email: ccf@pspawareness.com
2. **CurePSP**
   - Website: www.curepsp.org
   - Phone: 1-800-457-4777
   - Email: info@curepsp.org
3. **PSP Association**
   - Website: www.pspassociation.org.uk
   - Phone: +44 (0) 30 0111 4005
   - Email: helpline@pspassociation.org.uk
4. **National Institute of Neurological Disorders and Stroke (NINDS)**
   - Website: www.ninds.nih.gov
   - Phone: 1-800-352-9424
5. **American Academy of Neurology (AAN)**
   - Website: www.aan.com
   - Phone: 1-800-879-1960
6. **Parkinson's Foundation**
   - Website: www.parkinson.org
   - Phone: 1-800-4PD-INFO (473-4636)

References

This provides a comprehensive list of sources and further reading materials used in the creation of this guide. These references offer additional information and research on Progressive Supranuclear Palsy (PSP) for those interested in exploring the topic further.

Books

1. "The PSP Chronicles" by Tim Brown

Journal Articles

1. Smith, A. L., & Jones, B. R. (2020). Advances in the diagnosis and treatment of Progressive Supranuclear Palsy. *Journal of Neurology*, 267(3), 567-578.
2. Taylor, C. R., & Brown, M. E. (2019). Managing motor symptoms in Progressive Supranuclear Palsy: A review of current therapies. *Movement Disorders*, 34(5), 701-712.

Websites

1. CCF for PSP Awareness: www.pspawareness.com
2. CurePSP: www.curepsp.org
3. PSP Association: www.pspassociation.org.uk
4. National Institute of Neurological Disorders and Stroke (NINDS): www.ninds.nih.gov
5. American Academy of Neurology (AAN): www.aan.com
6. Parkinson's Foundation: www.parkinson.org

Research Databases

1. PubMed: Comprehensive resource for medical research articles.
2. ClinicalTrials.gov: Database of privately and publicly funded clinical studies conducted around the world.

Disclaimer

The information provided in this guide is intended for educational and informational purposes only. It is not a substitute for professional medical advice, diagnosis, or treatment. Always seek the advice of your physician or other qualified health provider with any questions you may have regarding a medical condition.

1. **Consult with Healthcare Providers:**
    - Always consult with a healthcare provider for medical advice tailored to your individual circumstances.
    - Do not disregard or delay seeking professional medical advice because of something you have read in this guide.
2. **Individual Variability:**
    - The management and treatment of PSP can vary widely among individuals.
    - What works for one person may not be suitable or effective for another.
3. **Updates and Advances:**
    - Medical knowledge and practices are constantly evolving.
    - Ensure you are accessing the most current information by consulting medical professionals and reputable sources regularly.
4. **Third-Party Resources:**
    - This guide references third-party websites, books, and other resources for additional information.
    - The inclusion of these references does not imply endorsement or guarantee of the accuracy of the information provided by these sources.
5. **No Liability:**
    - The authors, contributors, and publishers of this guide are not responsible for any adverse effects or consequences resulting from the use of any suggestions, treatments, or practices described in this guide.

Individual Profile

Personal Information	
Name:	
Date of Birth:	
Diagnosis Date:	
Primary Caregiver:	
Emergency Contact:	

Medical Information

Medical Team	
Neurologist:	
Primary Care Physician:	
Speech-Language Pathologist:	
Physical Therapist:	
Occupational Therapist:	

Symptoms and Progression

Symptoms	Severity (Mild, Moderate, Severe)
Bradykinesia (Slowness of Movement)	
Rigidity (Muscle Stiffness)	
Postural Instability (Balance Issues)	
Supranuclear Gaze Palsy (Eye Issues)	
Dysarthria (Speech Difficulties)	
Dysphagia (Swallowing Difficulties)	
Cognitive Changes	
Behavioral Changes	
Pain and Discomfort	

Medications

Medication	Dosage	Frequency	Notes
Medication	Dosage	Frequency	Notes

Therapies and Interventions

Therapy/Intervention	Frequency	Therapist/Provider
Physical Therapy		
Speech Therapy		
Occupational Therapy		
Palliative Care		

Daily Routine and Care Plan

Time	Activity	Notes
7:00 AM		
8:00 AM		
9:00 AM		
10:00 AM		
11:00 AM		
12:00 PM		
1:00 PM		
2:00 PM		
3:00 PM		
4:00 PM		
5:00 PM		
6:00 PM		
7:00 PM		
8:00 PM		

Emergency Information

Condition	Action	Emergency Contact
Choking	Perform Heimlich Maneuver/Call 911	
Severe Fall	Call 911	
Unconsciousness	Call 911	
Severe Pain	Administer Prescribed Pain Relief/Call 911	

NOTES

NOTES

NOTES

NOTES

NOTES

NOTES

NOTES

NOTES

NOTES

NOTES

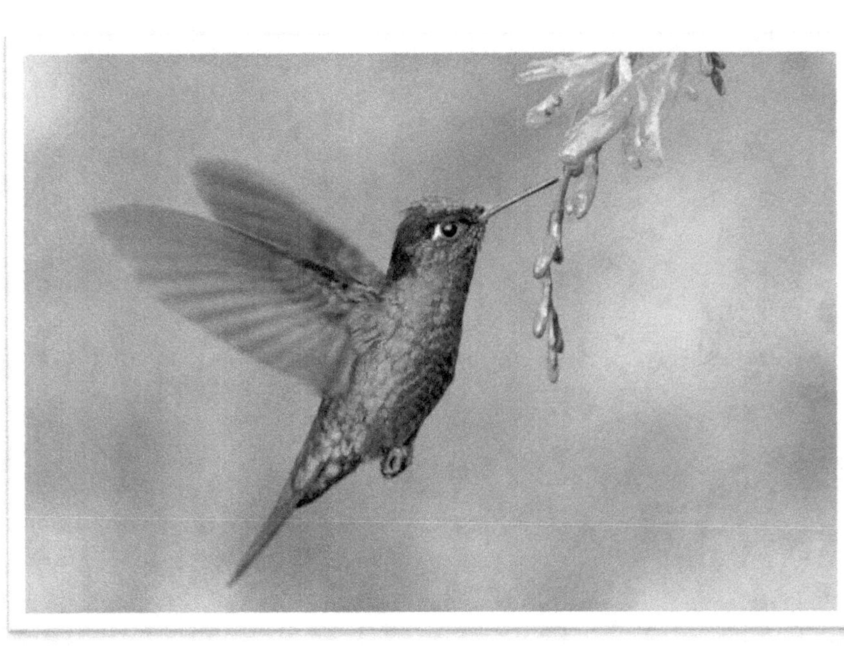

NO ONE WALKS ALONE

"Strength grows in the moments when you think you can't go on,
but you keep going anyway."

Laura Louizos